Fitness Tracking

Discover How To Improve Your Health
With
Fitness Tracking Technology Today

RON KNESS

Contents

Chapter 1: What is Health Tracking? And Why Should You Care?

If you haven't heard of fitness tracking, then you've probably been living under some kind of health *rock* for the past several years. Also known as health tracking, or life logging, fitness tracking is all about the 'quantified self'. In other words, it's about measuring your performance and your stats throughout the day as you train and as you go through your usual activities. This means things like your steps taken, heartrate, calories burned, temperature, stress levels and more.

Together, all this information can be combined to create a somewhat-complete picture of your health. You can then take that information and use it to guide your future training, to see where your weaknesses lie and hopefully to further improve your wellbeing.

The old maxim goes: 'that which is measured, improves'. This applies in business, it applies in engineering and yes, it applies in health and fitness.

In fact, there are some studies that suggest *simply measuring* your weight is enough to ensure you shed fat. That's right: with no other (conscious) changes to your lifestyle whatsoever, just knowing how much you weigh can help you to weigh less.

And it goes beyond that too. The more you learn about your fitness, the better you'll be able to improve your training methods and the more likely you are to be able to flag health problems and issues with your routine. It can be highly motivating to see yourself improve and it can provide data that allows you to train more efficiently and easily.

Using a fitness tracker for instance will let you train within your 'fat burning zone' and thereby burn fat far more efficiently than you otherwise would. Likewise, it will give you actionable tips on how to improve your sleep, thereby helping you to wake up with more energy.

Of course the reason that fitness tracking is so popular right now is partly to do with the slew of new technology now available that revolves around the tech. There are a huge number of wearable gadgets that provide fitness tracking, including the likes of the Microsoft Band 2, the Fitbit, Jawbone, the Garmin Vivofit, Apple Watch, Samsung Galaxy Gear Fit, the TomTom Spark and a plethora of other options.

If you really want to start tracking your health and improving your fitness, then picking any one of these gadgets can help you to do just that. At the same time though, there are also a number of different ways to measure your fitness and track your health that have *nothing* to do with wearable technology. People have been tracking their fitness and their performance for hundreds of years and there's no reason to spend lots of money on fancy wrist watches to do the same.

What *is* crucial is that you understand how to get the most out of fitness tracking, how to avoid some of the pitfalls and how to do it *right*. There's more than one way to go about measuring your health and fitness and if you take the wrong approach, you'll find that you end up ruining your own chances of success.

With the right skills and knowhow, you can track your progress with or *without* a fitness watch and the result will be better fat loss, more muscle, better sleep and more energy. Sound good?

That's where this book comes in.

What You Will Learn

In this book we'll be looking at a ton of different aspects revolving around fitness tracking. There aren't many books dedicated specifically to life logging which is a shame because there's just so much *to* it.

Within this text, you'll learn…

- ✓ How to pick the right fitness tracking options for you

- ✓ How to track calories

- ✓ How to work out your resting metabolic rate and active metabolic rate

- ✓ The best ways to measure fat and differentiate it from muscle

- ✓ How to measure your grip strength

- ✓ How to monitor your testosterone levels

- ✓ How to train in the fat burning zone

- ✓ How to use HIIT with a running watch

- ✓ How to calculate and compare your strength

- ✓ How to improve your brain with brain training

- ✓ How to increase your motivation with 'gamification'

- ✓ How to **guarantee** weight loss

✓ And MUCH more!

Chapter 2: The Top Fitness Trackers and Apps Available Today

In the introduction, we discussed how it wasn't actually necessary to were a 'fitness tracker' per se in order to effectively track your health and fitness. That is indeed true.

Nevertheless though, a fitness tracker *can* still do an awful lot to make life easier for you when you're monitoring your health and fitness. As the name would suggest, these devices are *all about* the fitness tracking and therefore should offer a more comprehensive overview of your health in one place than any other device or method.

A fitness tracker doesn't need to be expensive. In fact, it might only set you back $50 in some cases. This should be a *great* investment though as it will keep your health and fitness at the forefront of your mind and help you to learn much more about yourself in the process.

This chapter is your guide to picking the *right* fitness tracker.

What is a Fitness Tracker and What Should it be Able to do?

A good place to start is by asking what a fitness tracker is, what it does and what you should be looking for when you pick one.

To summarise then, a fitness tracker is any device that you wear on your person and that tracks some aspect of your fitness. To classify as a fitness tracker though, the device probably needs to have more than one function, or a 'smart element' such as the ability to sync with a smartphone or upload data to the cloud.

Many fitness trackers also offer a screen, which makes it easier for you to access the information and to use the device in other ways – though some you interact with *solely* through an app.

Most fitness trackers are worn on the wrist like a watch/bracelet, though there is a fair amount of variation here too. Some devices like the original Fitbit are instead worn on the belt, or as a new way I just saw, on the shoelace of the shoe. There are also some other interesting models in the works, which include one (called 'Jabra') that you wear inside the ears.

The most basic function that pretty much *every* fitness tracker out there offers then is a pedometer. Take your regular pedometer, give it a mobile app and you have your basic fitness tracker.

Most then use their in-built app in order to calculate other interesting data about you. In order to monitor steps, a pedometer needs to be able to measure movement and that means that it can roughly calculate your calories burned based on your activity (as long as you give it some basic information when you first set it up).

On top of the basic pedometer functionality, most trackers will include a gyroscope and accelerometer in order to measure more information about your movement. With a smart algorithm, a tracker can then deduce which activities you're engaged in and recognize if you're swimming or if you're cycling. More often, this technology is used to measure when you're sleeping – and how much you move during the night. This then allows for some basic sleep monitoring so that you can see how much deep sleep you're getting and how you might improve in order to feel more refreshed each morning.

From there, you then start to get a little more advanced with additional sensors. Galvanic skin response (GSR) is used to monitor whether or not a band is being worn. Another feature which is becoming more common is heart rate monitoring. Heart rate monitoring used to be achievable only with a chest strap (the most popular commercial option being those from Polar).

Today though, heartrate monitoring is possible through wrist-worn devices using infrared sensors which effectively film the pulsation of the veins. Some fitness trackers provide constant heartrate tracking, while others need to have that feature switched on during workouts.

Either way, the reliability of these readings is somewhat variable, which is something we'll be looking at more. An alternative offering comes from the UP3 from Jawbone. This device does away with the normal heartrate sensor and instead offers a 'bioimpedance sensor' which measures the resistance offered by the skin. This feature is actually very similar to how a treadmill works using the grips to monitor your heartrate.

Other features include temperature monitoring, GPS tracking (for runs) and even UV sensitivity. Which of these you need will of course depend on what you plan on monitoring.

A final important element for a lot of fitness trackers is the social element. Most fitness trackers allow you to compete with friends and relatives to see which of you are getting the most exercise and they allow you to compare yourself to other people in your demographic area. All this offers encouragement and support which can be a great help when you're struggling for motivation to get out and get training.

With all this in mind then, you should have a good picture of what a typical fitness tracker can offer. Let's move on to comparing a few of the top offerings to see how they hold up.

The Top Fitness and Activity Trackers

The Microsoft Band 2

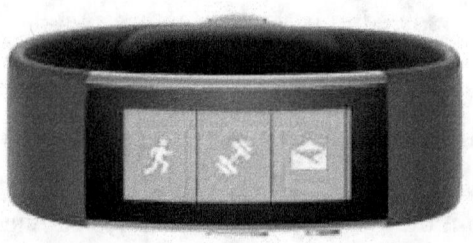

Let's start with a fitness tracker that sits at the top-end in terms of capabilities. While the Microsoft Band 2 (http://amzn.to/1RdjaMZ) is not the rock star of fitness tracking that Fitbit is, it nevertheless packs in a lot more sensors and features, and is potentially the most complete offering for those who are really keen on measuring their health.

With the Microsoft Band 2, you get the following sensors:

➤ All day LED heartrate monitoring
➤ Pedometer
➤ Accelerometer
➤ Gyroscope
➤ Microphone
➤ UV sensor

- ➢ GPS
- ➢ Barometer
- ➢ Ambient light sensor
- ➢ Galvanic skin response
- ➢ Temperature monitor

Together, these provide a truly comprehensive picture of your health. When you view the stats through the app or on your computer, you can how your heart rate changed throughout the day and how things like caffeine and sleep might have affected it. You can also see the number of steps you took, when you were most accurate and how many flights of stairs you ascended. You'll also see your calories burned of course.

Is the heart rate monitoring accurate? Overall the answer is yes. A Polar chest strap will still be *more* accurate but for most people it's not going to be far off. Your mileage may vary though and it appears that some factors like skin pigmentation may affect just how good a reading you get.

When you sleep, you get to see how long you slept versus how long you were in bed, how many times you woke up and how your heartrate varied throughout the night. Eventually, you'll start getting some contextual tips and advice on how to improve your sleep along with some 'observations'. The Band 2 also comes with a smart alarm which works by buzzing when you're at the lightest stages in your sleep up to 30 minutes before you set your alarm. This reduces 'sleep inertia' so you're not groggy when you get up.

When you train either in the gym or out running, you'll get an even more minute-by-minute breakdown of your heartrate. During training you'll be able to see how many calories you burned, how much of that was fat vs carbs, and what the 'cardio benefit' of that training was. With time, the Band can even tell you roughly what your VO2 max is, which a great measure of cardio fitness is.

If you're running and you turn on the GPS, you'll be able to see your routes mapped and a breakdown of your best speeds, splits, pace and times. Oh and using the UV sensor, it can tell you when it's time to put on sun cream!

What makes the Band 2 an improvement on the likes of Fitbit though is the big touchscreen which offers an intuitive and pleasant-to-use screen for getting around. This shows you data such as your current heartrate and pace when you're training but it also allows for more interesting things. For example, you can actually download pre-set workouts from the Microsoft Health App and then get talked through sets and reps or particular fitness drills. You can also create your own plans, which is a really nice touch.

There's even a 'golf' mode that tracks your performance on the golf course, measuring swings and practice swings and showing your route as you follow the holes around.

And better yet is the fact that the Microsoft Band 2 *also* works as a smartwatch. Not only does it allow you to see your messages, respond to them, read e-mails and check the weather – it also allows you install apps that others have made. Some of these are really useful, such as the 'music control' app that lets you control Spotify on your phone. These features actually have health benefit too – in that they prevent you from getting out your phone every two minutes and allow you to be more 'present' as a result.

The Microsoft Band 2 works on Android, iOS, Windows Phone and even Windows 10 for PC. The downside? It's about the most uncomfortable fitness tracker out there and can actually be a little tricky to sleep with. The first Band had some build quality issues and it's not waterproof so it's not a good option for swimmers. Battery life is also only 2 hours or less if you use the HR tracking, GPS or 'watch mode'.

TomTom Spark

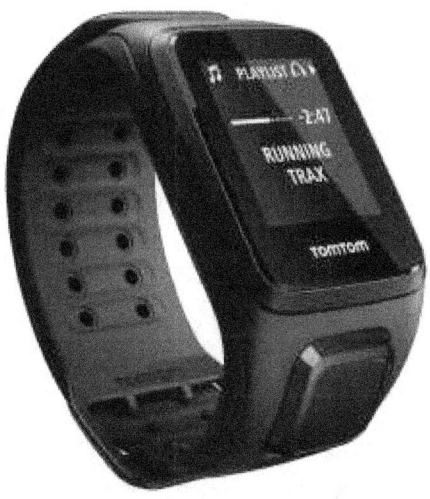

The TomTom Spark (http://amzn.to/1UyuiHW) is another top-end fitness tracker that has some real killer features. Compared with the Microsoft Band 2 it's not quite so pretty to look at but it's also a lot more comfortable. In terms of features, it also lacks the 'smartwatch' aspects of the Band 2 but makes up for it in the fitness features.

Sure, the TomTom Spark lacks a few of the Band 2's metrics like the barometer or the ability to calculate VO2 max. However, where it gets more useful is in the 5 day battery life and the waterproofing. These are great features for those who are really serious about tracking their fitness full time.

What's also cool about this option is that it provides you with the option to 'pick and choose' the features you want. Some models for instance will let you store music *on* the device (something else the Band can't do) so you don't have to take your phone on runs (you'll need Bluetooth headphones).

You can also optionally choose GPS tracking and heart rate monitoring and if you go for the full feature set, this will again be one of the most comprehensive trackers available. What's also cool is that you can use the Spark with a chest strap for more accurate readings.

Fitbit Surge

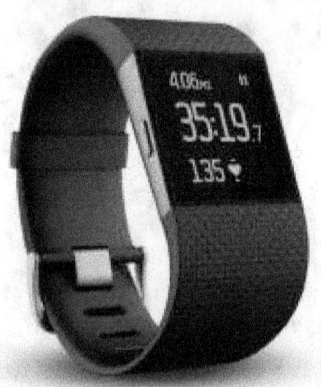

The latest Fitbit is the Surge (http://amzn.to/1UJlUnX). The feature set is very similar to that of the Spark with a heartrate monitor, pedometer, sleep tracking and a nice big display. It's not a smartwatch though, so you won't be using it to send texts or catch-up on Twitter. Unfortunately it isn't waterproof (like the Spark) but it does have GPS built-in.

Fitbit has one of the best apps from any fitness tracker and has been in the game long enough to build up a massive ecosystem. It syncs with a ton of different apps and has perhaps the very best social elements of any brand.

Like the Spark, the Surge has only a black and white display – whereas the Band 2, Apple Watch and Gear Fit all have colour touchscreens.

The odd thing is that the Fitbit Surge is actually more expensive than the Band 2 or some versions of the Spark despite doing less. If you're not fussed about the heartrate monitoring though, you could go with a different model of the Fitbit – such as the Flex – and that would also mean rocking a slightly more subtle look without the display (just a few lights). The Charge HR meanwhile offers you a tiny screen, plus heartrate monitoring – so again you can really pick the model that best suits you.

Jawbone UP3

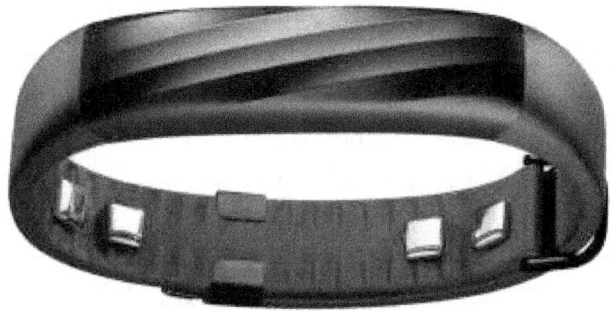

The Jawbone UP3 (http://amzn.to/1Uyv47T) is something completely different from the other options on this list. The Jawbone UP3 has *no* display which some people will see as a downside but other people will love.

Certainly the UP, UP24 and UP3 are sporting some of the most stylish designs of any fitness tracker and this is great if you want to carry on wearing a watch or if you want to avoid being too ostentatious with your technology. Jawbone is *also* one of the best options for women as its slim enough to fit around a thin wrist/arm and also has available designs that don't look like a big hulking piece of technology on your wrist.

The UP3 had lots of delays at launch which damaged its reputation. However, the heartrate tracking is interesting (though it offers snapshots throughout the day rather than continuous updates) and you do get some metrics you won't find anywhere else – like temperature during sleep.

There are other UP models too. The UP24 has no bioimpedance

More Options

We could go on forever, but the above should help to provide more than enough option.

In case you're still shopping for that perfect tracker though, you might also consider the **Nike Fuleband SE** (http://amzn.to/1ZkNoRq) which is great for gamification and which measures 'fuel points' rather than steps (which correspond to general activity). Otherwise this one is a basic monitor.

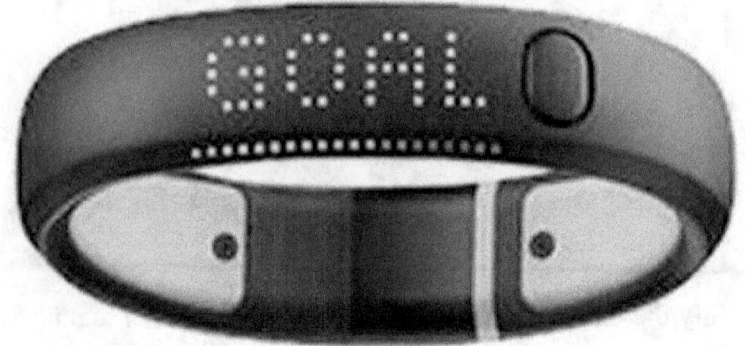

The **Basis Peak** (http://amzn.to/1ZkNoRq) is another cool one with temperature monitoring, smart exercise detection and HR.

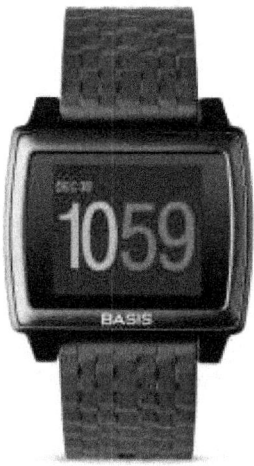

The **Gear Fit** (http://amzn.to/1T4dcR8) is a bit old now but has a (non 24 hour) heart rate sensor and a ton of smartwatch features relying on Android Wear.

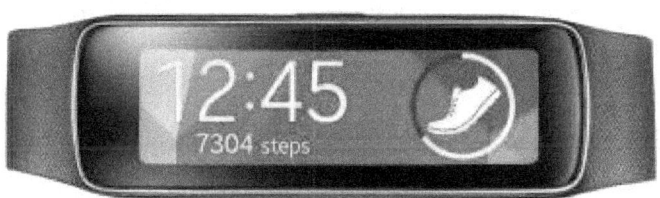

The **VivoSmart** (http://amzn.to/1UywZJs) from Garmin is a sleek fitness tracker which display that stays hidden until it needs to show a notification – and with a great price point. The **Vivosmart HR** (http://amzn.to/1T4dtng) adds heartrate monitoring.

The **Apple Watch** (http://amzn.to/1T4e5sR) also has a ton of health tracking features, though these are fairly light and the battery life is quite poor. If you like having the latest gadgets though and you are just looking for some entry level fitness tracking, then the **Apple Watch** will be a great way to get started.

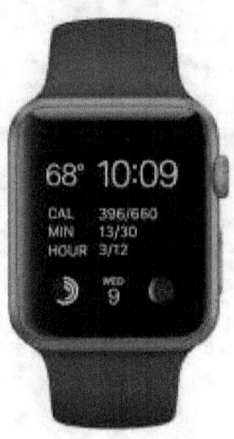

Then there are the weirder and less well-known options. The **Jabra Sport Pulse** (http://amzn.to/1MxC5Ol) measures your heartrate through your ears for instance and offers quite accurate data. There are also a whole plethora of different and strange fitness trackers on the way and already in the store, some of which we'll be looking at in the next section.

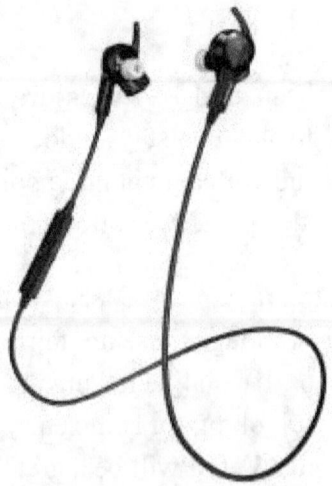

Phones

Note as well that a lot of phones have basic fitness tracking capabilities these days too. For example, the Galaxy Note 4 and 5 or the S4, 5 and 6 will both measure your heartrate, as do the latest iPhones. Almost every phone has a pedometer built in, or apps that can provide that function. There are also a ton of apps you can download that will further enhance the fitness tracking features of your devices. For example, you can download **MyRunKeeper (https://runkeeper.com/)** to track runs or **Endomondo (https://www.endomondo.com/)**, or you can use **MyFitnessPal (https://www.myfitnesspal.com/)** to track your calories. We'll look at these more in subsequent chapters.

Chapter 3: More Technology and Ways to Track Your Fitness

Let's imagine for a moment that you don't want to spend a ton of cash on any of the fancy fitness wearables we just looked at. That's fair enough, and probably quite sensible!

In this case, how would you track your fitness? Well… in a *ton* of different ways and as we'll see, you can certainly take a more MacGyver approach to this if that's more your style.

On the other end of the spectrum, if you want to get the most *complete* amount of information possible and you love being on the cutting edge of technology, then there are a ton of cool things you can do as well.

This chapter will look at some of the less conventional fitness tracking available – a lot of which also happens to be downright awesome…

Oh and some of these tracking methods are things that you need to be doing on top of using your fitness tracker anyway. In this section you'll learn how to calculate things like your BMR and AMR.

Old-School Fitness Tracking

Want to go old-school on your fitness tracking? Here are some basic utilities you can use…

Getting Your Heartrate

If you want to monitor your heartrate without a fitness tracking watch, then you have a few options. One is to go to a gym with treadmills and other cardio machines and then just to hold onto the handles. Normally, these will use bioimpedance sensors to give you a good reading and if you keep your training consistent and take note of your heart rate, you'll be able to see your fitness improve over time. Another option is to buy a **Polar chest strap (http://amzn.to/1ZkYS7y)**, which works with a lot of these machines and isn't too expensive.

Failing that, why not do things the old fashioned way and just take your pulse with your fingers? To do this, just take your fingers and place them on the inside of your wrist, right below your thumb. Count how many beats you can feel in 10 seconds (using a timer) and then multiply by 6 to get the result of your beats per minute (BPM).

To measure your resting heartrate, just take your pulse first thing in the morning. This gives you a good indicator of your overall cardio health (a healthier heart has to beat fewer times to circulate the same amount of blood) and also tells you how much you recovered during the night and whether or not you're ready to train again.

Measuring Your Weight

Something you should definitely be doing even if you wear the most advanced strap in the world is measuring your weight. This is an important metric to know generally but it's especially useful if you're trying to lose weight.

Now, it's important to be careful when measuring weight and using this along with dieting. The problem with measuring weight alone is that it doesn't differentiate between muscle and fat.

Weight alone is actually a fairly useless metric then because what's more important is body composition.

How do you measure this? One option is to submerge yourself in a special tank that can measure your mass via a clever displacement system… but you probably don't want to afford all that.

Instead, why not just measure your waistline? If you're looking to lose weight then no doubt this is basically what you're trying to affect and it will offer a much more useful number to base your training on.

BMR and AMR

We said that you needed to know your weight for general purposes too though and this is a good example of that. Your BMR and AMR can be used to tell you how many calories you burn in any given day but in order to know this number, you need your weight first.

When calculating your calories burned, any fitness tracker is going to first calculate your AMR and BMR based on some data you put in.

Essentially, your BMR is your 'Basal Metabolic Rate' which is the number of calories you burn when you're just lying there. You need to burn calories just in order to blink, in order to beat your heart and in order to breathe.

The AMR (Activity Metabolic Rate) meanwhile is the number of calories you burn based on your activity. That doesn't just mean fitness training but also things like walking, going to work, etc.

To calculate your basal metabolic rate, you use the following equations:

Men:

BMR = 66 + (6.23 x weight in pounds) + (12.7 x height in inches) – (6.8 x age in years)

Women:

BMR = 655 + (4.35 x weight in pounds) + (4.7 x height in inches) – (4.7 x age in years)

To turn this into your AMR, you then multiply that amount by:

> ➢ 1.2 if you're sedentary (little or no exercise)
> ➢ 1.375 if you're lightly active (you exercise 1-3 times a week)
> ➢ 1.55 if you're moderately active (you exercise or work about average)
> ➢ 1.725 if you're very active (you train hard for 6-7 days a week)
> ➢ 1.9 if you're highly active (you're a physical laborer or a professional athlete)

With this number, you'll then know how many calories you burn both before and after exercise. This is useful as it lets you know roughly how many calories you can consume before you're likely to start gaining weight. Moreover, it's important to keep in mind when reading how many calories you burned. Why? Because the exercise you're doing is only accounting for a small proportion of the extra calories. Saying you burned 200 calories in an hour is less impressive when you realize that you normally burn at least 83 calories in an hour anyway.

Strength

Want to measure your strength? There are a number of ways you can do this but one very simple one is to measure your 1 rep maximum on a variety of lifts – ideally the big three compound lifts (those being the squat, deadlift and bench press).

The problem with this plan is that a one rep max is quite hard to measure if you don't have a spotter. Something you can do though is to find a weight you can lift five times and then to use the following equation:

(5RM x 1.1307) + 0.6998

This is roughly the same no matter *what* type of exercise you're performing.

Another option is to measure the size of your muscles with tape measures. This is something that professional bodybuilders do a lot and it's a great way to see if you're gaining size in specific areas.

Of course muscle size does not correlate precisely with muscle strength for a variety of reasons and once again, there's no way to differentiate between fat here. Still, if size is what you're actually aiming for (as it is for a lot of guys) then this is the most logical thing to measure!

The Mirror

That said, another way to measure your aesthetics is quite simply to take a look in the mirror. As long as you're able to be objective, this is the easiest way to see where you have fat still clinging on, which muscles are looking the biggest/the most defined and where you can improve.

Take photos as you train and compare them with how you look in the mirror and make sure that you think about what is that you're doing that's causing the positive results or the lack thereof.

Pen and Paper

One of the best tools you can possibly use to measure your fitness and to track your performance though is a good old-fashioned pad of paper and a pen.

What can you monitor with this? That all depends on what you're trying to measure. One particularly good example though would be to just write down how you *feel* each morning on a scale of one-to-ten. From there, you can start tracking what you're eating, how you're training, what time you're going to bed etc. and then look for correlations. You might be able to find for instance that you feel bad on the days when you have too much caffeine, or on the days that you eat bread – maybe you have a gluten intolerance! The point is, that by keeping tabs on how you feel and what you're doing, you might be able to identify correlations that offer useful insights and help you to improve your health.

Tracking your workouts is also a good idea. Keep tabs on precisely what amounts you're lifting and how, where you're running etc. This way you can then compare that data to your stats and see whether all the hard work is really paying off.

There are also a ton of social networks that allow you to do this on a more public forum and here you can also benefit from some of the social benefits that something like Fitbit offers. For instance, **Body Space (http://bodyspace.bodybuilding.com/)** is a great site from Bodybuilding.com where you can share your progress, your goals and your pictures and get motivation and feedback from the community.

Health Checks

One more tip is to visit your doctor regularly for health checks. There doesn't need to be something wrong with you to see your GP – just ask for a blood test and your blood pressure to be monitored and you can keep tabs on your general fitness. If you have the money, then paying to see a physio occasionally can help you to avoid getting into bad posture habits and to prevent picking up bad movement habits. All these things give you more information and early warning of problems, which can make a *massive* difference to your health.

More Cool Fitness Tracking Devices

Are you loving all of this data tracking and learning that much more about your body? If so then you might be itching to put yourself right at the forefront of the field and to try some of the latest and most exciting products and options on the market. Here are some more advanced tools for the pro life-logger.

Dynamometer

Something pretty cheap that you can invest in to get a fun little insight into your health and fitness is a 'dynamometer'. This is basically a device that you squeeze with your grip as hard as you can and which then measures how much force you applied. In turn, this lets you tell how strong you are in terms of your grip (which has a huge correlation with your overall strength) and also gives you some feedback regarding your recovery. It's often said that a weak grip in the morning suggests that you have a low ratio of testosterone to cortisol and in turn this implies that you haven't recovered all that well from your last workout.

The **Dynamometer (http://amzn.to/1MxI1XR)** is also a great tool for training in itself as it offers you a way to test your grip strength that can go up to 90KG (unlike a lot of grip 'trainers').

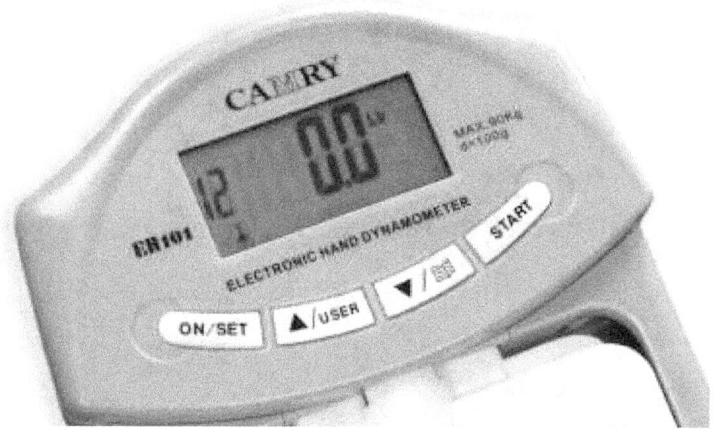

The Skulpt

The **Skulpt (http://amzn.to/1UfWNL2)** is a relatively new fitness tracking device that found popularity on Kickstarter. What it does is allow you to measure your muscle 'quality' which tells you the density of the muscle that you're working. It measures 12 different muscle groups and for those looking for something completely unique and original, this is a fun metric to measure.

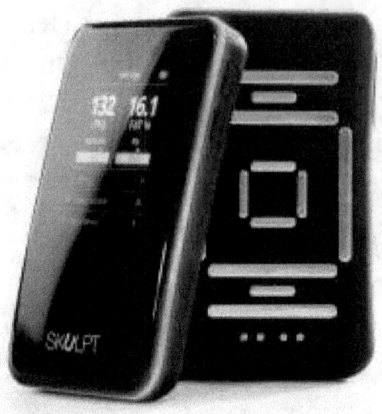

Cue

The Cue health tracker is device that is currently still in development but which promises to revolutionize health tracking by allowing you to take readings from your blood from home. These include vitamin D (which many of us are deficient in), inflammation, influenza, fertility and testosterone. For many guys and especially gym rats, the testosterone measurement will be the one here that's most interesting and this can be a great tool if you're trying to improve your anabolism through lifestyle and diet.

Blood and DNA Tests

There are now a number of services online that offer some deeper insights into your health, such as blood analysis and even DNA tests. WellnessFX for instance is one such service that can measure 53-93 markers depending on what you're looking for, though the price is quite steep. Other sits like DNAFit offer DNA testing for fitness and other uses. These can tell you things about yourself such as your ratio of slow twitch to fast twitch muscle fiber – useful insights that will help you to pick the right style of training to see the fastest results.

This isn't a requirement by any stretch of the imagination and you shouldn't waste your money on it if you haven't started seeing progress already. But if you have the cash spare and you find that your interest in fitness tracking is more than just a phase, then collecting this kind of data can help you to build the most truly comprehensive picture of your health possible.

Unusual Fitness Trackers

In the future, we'll see a range of fitness trackers that do incredible things. Some are available already. FitLinxx for instance is an interesting tracker that sticks to your skin and measures some unique metrics. More impressive are things like the **Atlas Wristband (http://amzn.to/1WD6UXQ)** for measuring precise exercises. This one can tell when you're doing specific movements and count your sets and reps – things like dumbbell curls and deadlifts are all automatically registered by the device. This is a potential game changer for people in the gym and for the aforementioned weight lifting tracking.

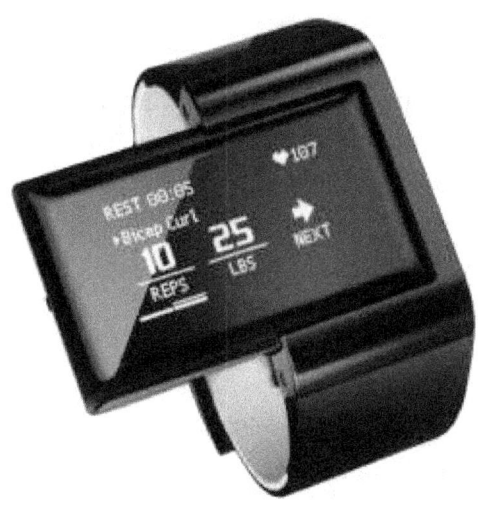

Another game changer for gym nuts? The incredible GymWatch (http://amzn.to/1RwTfgj). This is a device that can actually measure raw *strength* by measuring your movement and comparing this with some information you input regarding the weight you're going to be lifting.

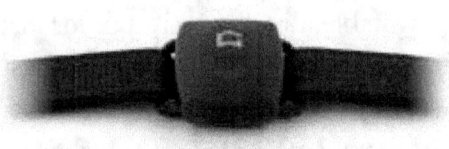

Pavlock goes an entirely different route and focuses on preventing you from breaking your goals and resolutions. How? By delivering a short and sharp electric shock!

You can also find 'smart toothbrushes' that monitor exactly how long you spend brushing and point out which teeth you've missed. Then there's the somewhat creepy 'mother' from 'Sen.se' which watches everything you do and monitors all kinds of habits like whether or not you wash your hands.

In other words, if you think that a tracker should exist then there's a good chance it's out there. These devices aren't *just* for measuring your ability to run or how many calories you burn. You can track everything from your tooth brushing habits to your DNA!

Chapter 4: Using Apps and Trackers to Fix Your Diet

So far this is all very exciting but we've yet to see how any of it can be used to accomplish any real results.

All that changes here though. Let's start with diet: how can you use all this data in order to improve your diet and *guarantee* weight loss? Because you really can guarantee weight loss when you get serious about health tracking. This isn't hyperbole and it isn't any fancy new fad – it's just simple math.

How Health Tracking Guarantees Weight Loss

Basically, fat loss comes down to one simple rule: in order to lose weight and burn fat, you need to make sure that you burn more calories than you consume.

Therefore, if you are burning off more calories than you're taking in, you *will* create a deficit and you *will* start to get slimmer, more toned and more lean.

Now at this point, some people might be tempted to point out that 'not all calories are made equal' or that they can also lose weight by keeping their blood sugar levels down.

Is that true?

Well, that massively depends on who you ask. It probably *is* true that not all the calories you consume reach your blood and things like the 'thermogenic effect' do play a role. But the impact of these factors is also likely to be very small. And they're even *smaller* when you compare them to the *huge* impact of calories.

No matter what else is true, if you eat fewer calories than you burn then you will lose fat. Simple, straightforward and non-negotiable.

So with that in mind, there are just a few metrics you need to record to absolutely guarantee that you lose weight:

- ➢ Your BMR and BMA (see last chapter)
- ➢ Your caloric intake
- ➢ Your exercise

Tools for Tracking Calories

When it comes to tracking the calories that you're eating, you can use a large number of different apps. **MyFitnessPal** is one of the most popular options and will sync up with a ton of apps like Microsoft's Health App for the Band 2. When you combine this data, you can then see how many calories are coming in, how many are being burned and what the difference is.

Otherwise, you can also use apps that come with various fitness trackers. S Health is available for Samsung devices and the Gear Fit, while Microsoft Health also has calorie monitoring capabilities.

To measure your caloric intake, you simply need to look at the back of your food and find the 'Kcal'. This means 'Kilo Calorie' and is what most of us are referring to when we measure calories. Each time you eat something, check out the calories (you can ask in restaurants and look on websites belonging to cafes and takeaways) and then input the amount you consumed. In some cases, apps will have the calories for the food you consume already inputted by another user and that means you only need to find it from a list. Things you eat regularly will find their way to the top of the list and you can then add their calories easily with a swipe and a tap.

Meanwhile, you can use a device with 24 hour heartrate monitoring such as the Microsoft Band 2 or the TomTom Spark in order to get an accurate reading of how many calories you burned. If you don't have one of those, then you can just look at your AMR for a rough average.

Now you might find that you typically eat 2,300 calories and burn 2,000 (2,000 is an average AMR for most of us). What this means is that you have a 'surplus' of 300 calories at the end of each day and where do you think that goes? That's right: it's stored as fat.

Meanwhile, if you consume 1,700 calories and manage to burn 2,300 now you have a deficit of 600 calories. This means your body will need to *burn* fat just to make it through the day and you'll lose weight. A 3,500 weekly calorie deficit results in a one pound loss. That breaks down into a 500 calorie per day deficit.

As you collect more data, you can then look at what you are eating that's adding the most calories and how much fat you're burning typically through your training.

What you'll find is that some clear ways to shift the balance present themselves. Forget that cappuccino or swap it for an Americano on the way to work and you just saved yourself 100 calories. Get off a bus stop earlier and powerwalk into work and you just burned an extra 100 calories. That's 200 calories back which might just be enough to help you start losing weight again.

Likewise, you can also see what's working in the gym. Maybe you notice you burn more calories when you're hitting the heavy bag instead of running. Simple solution? Hit the heavy bag longer.

Logging your health is what makes it possible for you to approach this change in a scientific, bulletproof manner. A fitness tracker isn't necessary, though it will help you to see which parts of your day are particularly good or bad for you in terms of calories burned.

How to Change Your Calories Without the Headache

With the best app in the world, logging your calories is still unfortunately a massive headache that takes up a lot of time and effort.

There is one device that promises to measure your calories automatically by measuring glucose levels in your cells. That's the Healbe Gobe. Unfortunately, most reviewers conclude that this technology doesn't quite work yet – but it's promising that might be on the horizon someday. For now? Sadly a lot of professionals believe that this type of calorie measuring is just simply *impossible*.

So back to the problem at hand: how do you measure the calories you're eating without letting it drive you completely mad?

One option is to take a more 'general' approach.

Try this…

Monitor your caloric intake for a few days. Look at things you eat *regularly* – for instance maybe you have the same cereal every morning or a pretty consistent lunch. If you don't? Well then maybe it's time that you started! Eating consistently makes it much easier to track your calories as well as to find a routine that works for you.

Now what you do is simply looking for the biggest calorie culprits that you can cut out or swap. If that chocolate cereal is full of sugar then you might just want to swap it with something a little plainer such as some oatmeal.

Likewise you can swap out your soda drink for water – this is an area where a lot of calories tend to sneak in under the radar.

Of course your dinners are going to vary but if your breakfast and lunch are *fairly* consistent then you'll know how many calories you have left to 'spend' come the evening. This then means that you can simply try to avoid consuming anything that will represent a massive calorie dump.

For me it was pizza. I never realized – until I took the time to look – that the pizzas I ate often contained 500-700 calories. As my AMR is 2,200, that was a massive amount for me to spend on dinner! Pie and chips night was even worse…

So the solution was just to cut those out or at least to eat them a lot less often – really simple. And if I knew I was having them that night? Then that was a great time to go for a 6 mile run which would burn me 700-800 calories. You see how this works?

The point here is that it doesn't have to be precise or exact – just measure enough to get a general idea and then afford yourself a *little* flexibility to try and avoid driving yourself completely insane.

Another thing to consider in respect to all of this is that there is no way that you can *possibly* learn your exact calorie intake or burn. It's just too varied – of course there are different numbers of calories in apples for example! And likewise, your testosterone fluctuates every single day, which in turn has a big impact on your ability to burn calories.

So don't try and track it precisely. Track is *generally* and aim to consume about 500 calories less than you burn (while your aim is weight loss). If you manage this, then you'll be able to consistently burn fat and even when you make a mistake, you still won't go over your calorie burn.

Of course it's also super important to be careful *what* you eat and to make sure you're fuelling your body with all the crucial vitamins, minerals, amino acids and other nutrients that you need. That's a topic for an entirely different book though and a whole subject onto itself.

Chapter 5: How to Get the Most Out of Fitness Tracking for Training

So now you know how to use your fitness tracking in order to burn fat and improve your diet: know the calories in and the calories out and then sway them in your favor. Sorted.

Likewise, you know how to use fitness tracking to just *feel* better: you keep a log of all your activities, your diet and your habit and then make regular notes of how you feel. Look for correlations and you're golden.

But what about training and working out? How do you use fitness trackers to improve your effectiveness in that domain?

Staying in the Fat Burning Zone

One very useful tool for training that presents itself once you start tracking your fitness and your training is the optimum 'fat burning zone'.

The fat burning zone is a somewhat controversial topic, as some people will claim that it doesn't exist. Is this true? Well yes and no. The argument really surrounds the perfect pace at which you should be training in order to burn the maximum amount of fat and while some people say you need to train *more* intensively, other people say you should train *less* intensively.

The level that most people tell you to train is at 75% of your MHR. MHR is 'Maximum Heart Rate' and to get this figure, you just need to take your tracker, heart rate monitor or CV machine of choice and then train as intensively as you can (while remaining safe).

You'll find that your data shows the point at which you peaked and if you take that number, that is your MHR. 75%, according to many, is your optimum fat burning zone and the zone at which you should try to stay within when training in order to shed pounds.

Interestingly though, it seems that a higher level of intensity is going to be more useful for burning the maximum number of calories. Note here the distinction between calories and fat.

You see, it all comes down to the way in which your body burns the calories. When you work out at above 75% of your MHR, you enter an 'anaerobic' type of training, which means that you'll need energy more quickly than your body can burn it for fuel. That means that the only source of energy is the glucose in the blood and at this point you've then stopped burning fat and started burning carbs.

But that doesn't mean that high intensity training is useless. Because once you *exit* that high intensity training, your body will *then* start to get more of its energy from your fat stores because it has nowhere else to look. This means you actually burn more calories overall and more *fat* in the long-term because you change the metabolism of your body.

What counts as high intensity training? That's about 90-95% of your MHR.

But of course not everyone is going to want to train at 90-95% of their capacity as it will pose health risks if you're elderly or if you have heart problems. For those who are willing to go intense, the next section on HIIT will sort you out. For everyone else, training in the 70-80% range is still useful and will still burn lots of calories.

Either way, taking a look at your wrist will let you know how heart your body is working and whether you need to increase the intensity or lower it.

HIIT

Even if you *are* super athletic, you won't be able to maintain anaerobic exercise for long before you collapse. That's why the marathon isn't sprinted by anyone but rather jogged.

What you *can* do though, is to use interval training. This means that you'll be alternating between periods of high intensity and lower intensity. So you might train at 90% of your MHR for about 2 minutes and then drop down to 70% for 5 minutes while you recover.

What's excellent about this strategy is that it allows you to burn more calories in less time without killing yourself. At the same time, it also means that you can use *both* strategies for burning fat. This is great because it means that you use the anaerobic type of training in order to remove your blood glucose and then immediately follow this up with lower intensity training to burn off the optimum amount of fat. It's a hugely efficient and scientific approach to your training and fitness tracking really makes this much easier.

(As an added bonus, HIIT also increases the efficiency of your mitochondria. We won't go into this in detail here, but suffice to say that your mitochondria handles your body's ability to utilize glucose for energy. The more you have and the more efficient they are, the more energetic you become and the more fat your body burns.)

Guided Workouts

Using the above strategies, you can use your fitness tracker in order to improve the efficiency of your workouts and to burn more calories.

If you're interested in doing HIIT, then look for a fitness tracker with guided workouts such as the Microsoft Band 2. It is particularly great for this because it includes some workouts for HIIT, etc. that will talk you through the training as you're doing it. This means you know exactly when to increase the tempo and when to lower it and you're never left guessing. You can even find programs over the course of several weeks, almost like having a personal trainer right there with you!

But what if you're less interested in burning calories and more interested in building muscle or improving your athletic performance? Guided workouts can help a ton with this too and can teach you the right techniques to use such as drop sets and supersets, while at the same time encouraging the correct form on things like the Deadlift.

As mentioned there's also the Atlas fitness tracker that promises to be able to monitor your actual technique and reps and sets and the GymWatch to measure strength. *Or* you can look at the **Moov Now** (http://amzn.to/1U534su) which also promises to be able to provide useful advice regarding technique via a voice in your ear and fitness tracking that monitors multiple limbs.

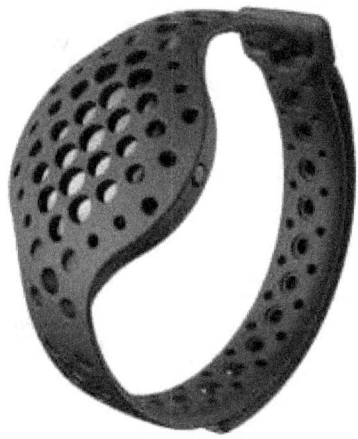

Another option is to use Xbox Fitness which will use the Kinect on Xbox One to analyse your actual movements – and potentially even combine this information with data from the Microsoft Band 2.

As mentioned though, simply keeping track of your regime and monitoring improvements in your strength can go a long way to telling you whether your current techniques and programming are working.

Recovery

Another vitally important metric/readout that your trackers should offer you relating to your training is your recovery. The best trackers and especially those designed with running in mind, will be able to tell you exactly how long you need to rest before you can train again. If you do a particularly intense workout for 1.5 hours, it might recommend you wait a few days.

HEED this warning. This is one of the biggest things that a lot of people get wrong when starting out in the gym: they train super hard for five days a week and they don't give their bodies time to recover. Remember, this is very often straight off the back of doing *nothing*. Unsurprisingly, they reach burnout after not long, which is more technically known as 'overtraining'. At that point, they then find themselves unable to make it to the gym at all anymore and they see all their enthusiasm fade.

Slow and steady wins the race. Listen to this recommendation.

Chapter 6: Fitness Tracking for Runs

Where fitness tracking *really* comes into its own though is when you strap on a pair of running shoes and head outside for a jog or a run.

In fact, if you've only ever run *without* a fitness tracker previously, you'll find that this completely changes the effectiveness of your training and you'll wonder how you ever survived before.

When using a fitness tracker on a run, you'll want to use it to measure several metrics:

> ➢ Your heartrate
> ➢ Distance
> ➢ Route
> ➢ Calories
> ➢ Time
> ➢ Pace
> ➢ Splits

To help you recognize what some of this means, your pace effectively tells you how fast you're going in terms of minutes for each mile or each kilometer. So the lower the score you have for your pace, the faster you're going.

Your split meanwhile is the time that you completed a specific mile. This is useful because it can show you how your performance improved or worsened over the duration of your run and it also lets you try and burn more calories in a set amount of time.

Of course knowing the distance you've run is also useful because it lets you aim for a specific target, which your calories and heartrate can also do.

Finally, with GPS switched on, you'll get more accurate readings for everything else and you'll also have the fun of being able to see precisely the route you took and the laps you made. This is not only useful, it's also just a bit of fun – if you ever go on holiday and go for a run while you're out there for instance, you'll be able to see logs your activity in other countries!

The Difference When Fitness Tracking

Depending on what you're trying to improve, you can aim for different scores and figures in different areas. For example, if your focus is purely on losing weight, then you can go for a run with the aim of burning X number of calories and just come home once you've done that. On the other hand, if you're training for the marathon, then you might be more interesting in watching your average pace and your splits. You can use this data in order to see how well you're performing and how quickly you're completing your different legs. You'll also know how to pace yourself for maximum performance across the distance.

More interested in improving fitness? Then keep your heartrate at a certain level and monitor the 'fitness benefit' suggestion and how your VO2 max is improving. All of this information is useful for running and it makes a *huge* difference.

Before fitness trackers, how would you go about using a run to get fit? Simple: you'd head out for a run, you'd jog randomly around a track or a large field and you'd come home when you were tired. Sure, you could use other tools like Endomondo or MyRunKeeper on their own, but this involves a lot more effort and work. If you are serious about running, then a fitness tracker with built-in GPS is a *very* good idea.

Chapter 7: The Dark Side of Fitness Tracking

As you can see then, fitness tracking can absolutely revolutionize your training. It does this by taking the kind of 'shotgun' approach you might be using at the moment and transforming it into a fine scalpel or a laser. You now use math and numbers to make sure you're getting the precise amount of exercise you need, that you're not eating too much and that you're training in the most efficient manner. You keep an eye on the numbers and you can know with certainty whether you're going to lose weight or not.

But there are downsides to fitness tracking too and you do need to be a *little* careful in some respects.

One pitfall for instance is the possibility that you end up reliant on your fitness tracking devices. This can then be a problem if your fitness device should break and you trust it whole heartedly. Imagine for instance that your device goes mad and starts telling you that you have a resting heartrate of 140bpm. You might now start worrying about your health, skipping the gym and potentially eating less carefully seeing as you'll probably be burning '10,000 calories a day'.

Of course no one has a resting BPM that high and in this case, it's more likely that your device is just damaged. What's key is that you recognize this possibility and don't just believe it.

The solution in this case? *Listen* to your body. Use your intuition and learn to feel what a high heart rate is like and what a low heart rate is like. If your fitness tracker is telling you one thing and your body is telling you another, check it by taking your pulse the old fashioned way!

A similar problem is what happens when you forget to wear your tracker or you miss a workout. Fitness tracking can be surprisingly addictive and this can make the whole process a little stressful if you occasionally miss a session.

One way to solve this problem is to use multiple tracking techniques. For instance, you might use Microsoft Health *and* S Health and combine the tracking of your Fitbit with the tracking of your phone. This way, when you forget to charge your device, you'll still be able to monitor your steps.

But likewise, try not to get too obsessive over your health tracking. This is a tool to serve a purpose. That purpose is all that matters – you don't need a complete data set and it's probably not going to be 100% accurate anyway!

Every now and then try taking a break from fitness tracking. You don't need it on holiday and it's good to stop monitoring yourself like a hawk once in a while.

Chapter 8: Conclusions – 5 More Tips for Better Fitness Tracking

And there you have it! Everything you possibly could need to know in order to start getting the best out of fitness tracking. Hopefully you've discovered some exciting new options you didn't know about when it comes to tracking your health and hopefully you now know how to start getting more from your diet, from your runs, from your weightlifting and more. Once you fall into a system that works for you and start collecting the data that matters to your goals, you'll be able to keep real tabs on what's happening in your body, whether you're losing weight and what you need to change in order to make positive progress.

Well, perhaps we haven't covered *everything*. I'll leave you with these five additional tips that can help you get even more from your tracking activities…

1 Choose Your Wrist

When you wear your tracker, make sure to tell it which wrist it is on. Most trackers have an option to do this and when you do, you'll get more accurate readings based on more accurate knowledge about the movements coming in.

2 Use it to Stay Calm

Fitness tracking has been around long before the Fitbit and is actually a powerful medical tool used by doctors and GPs. In this context, fitness tracking and heart rate monitoring in particular, are used to provide something called 'biofeedback'. Biofeedback basically means that you see information about your health such as your heartrate and/or blood pressure and thereby learn to identify certain symptoms in your body and even to control your heartrate.

Your fitness tracker thus can be used to help you improve your sense of calm. Keep an eye on your heartrate and focus on calming your mind. See if you can get your heartrate to slow down by thinking calm thoughts and concentrating.

3 Strengthen Your Brain Too!

Tracking is just for the body – it's for the mind as well! You can use exercises to train and track things like your attention, memory and reactions with the dual n-back test, or programs like **Lumosity** or **BrainHQ**. You can even get 'trackers' that help you monitor things like your ability to concentrate. The 'NeuroWave' is one of the first commercial devices to offer EEG readings and works with a smart app.

4 Start Small

Another potential pitfall when starting out with fitness and health tracking is that you risk overloading yourself with data and information. Start small and build up!

5 Use Gamification

Gamification means turning an objective into a game. A classic example of this would be to challenge yourself to burn an extra calorie every day and to award yourself some kind of badge or medal on a chart each time you do. When you approach challenges like this, they become a lot more fun and the small rewards provide you with constant encouragement and feedback. Gamification goes perfectly hand-in-hand with fitness tracking!

Well, that's enough theory to get you going – now comes the fun part: putting it into practice! Start tracking some small right now and build from there. You'll be amazed at how it can transform your life and improve your fitness and health across the board.

And of course this is just the beginning, the future holds *amazing* things for fitness tracking!

Other Senior Health and Fitness Books by This Author

If you would like to read more about Senior Health and Fitness, here is a list of the titles, CreateSpace links and descriptions:

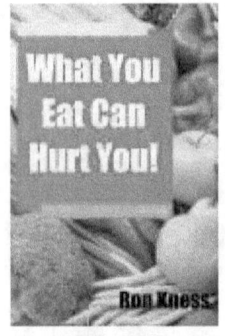

What You Eat Can Hurt You

https://www.createspace.com/4963196

Do you know that certain foods increase your risk for inflammation, disease and illness? It's true! And certain foods can help cure and heal you if you do get sick. Knowing which foods to eat and which ones to avoid empowers you to manage your own health.

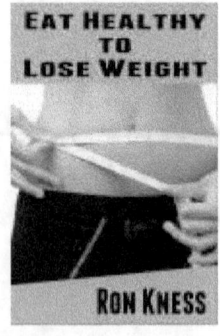

Eat Healthy to Lose Weight

https://www.createspace.com/4962939

As you read through our book, we show you which foods you should and should not be eating to reach your weight loss goal, along with discussing how to maintain your weight loss and stay within a few pounds of your goal weight. Banish the weight you keep gaining back each time by learning how to live a healthy lifestyle.

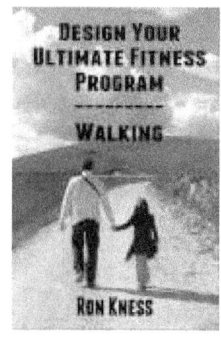

Design Your Ultimate Fitness Program - Walking

https://www.createspace.com/5252272

In my book Design Your Ultimate Fitness Program – Walking, we discuss the considerations that need to be made when designing a custom walking program, along with:
• Equipment needed
• Wearable technology you can use to track your walking
• And how to make walking more challenging

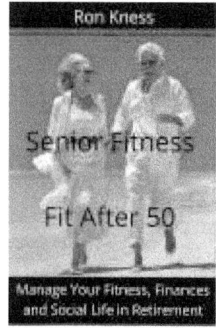

Senior Fitness – Fit After 50: Learn How to Manage Your Fitness, Finances and Social Life in Retirement

https://www.createspace.com/5474751

Inside you will discover answers to your most pressing questions:
• What do I need to know about downsizing my home?
• What are the best tips for staying healthy as you approach your 50's?
• When should I start planning for retirement?
• I am worried about being lonely once I retire, do others feel the same?
• Is it worthwhile to carry two homes during retirement?
And more…

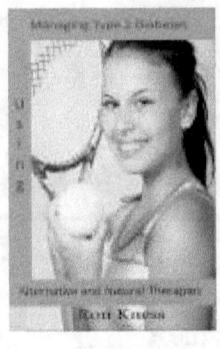

Managing Type 2 Diabetes Using Alternative And Natural Therapies

https://www.createspace.com/5401244

While Type 2 diabetes can be managed medically, there are many alternative natural and holistic methods of therapy and treatment that can further enhance quality of life and minimize the effects of this disease. In this book, I discuss 12 different types, including yoga, reflexology and acupuncture to name just three.

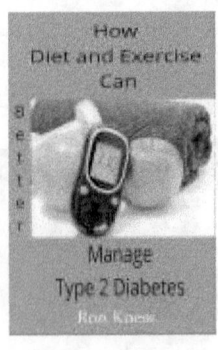

How Diet and Exercise Can Better Manage Type 2 Diabetes

https://www.createspace.com/5404845

Of the different types of diabetes, only Type 2 can be reversed. In my book How Diet and Exercise Can Better Manage Type 2 Diabetes, we reveal the three things you can do to best manage your disease, including:
• Diet
• Exercise
• Weight management

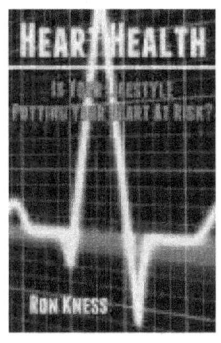

Heart Health: Is Your Lifestyle Putting Your Heart at Risk?

https://www.createspace.com/5464020

In my ebook Is Your Lifestyle Putting Your Heart At Risk? we discuss the six greatest risks to your heart and the lifestyle changes you can make to mitigate them.

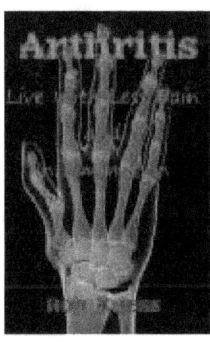

Arthritis – Live Wth Less Pain and Inflammation: Tips and Techniques You Can Use to Lessen the Pain and Inflammation

https://www.createspace.com/5457441

Discover Simple Tips & Information That Will Help Reduce The Painful Symptoms Of Arthritis!

You learn things like:
• Simple and effective information that will help you manage the pain and inflammation that comes along with arthritis, so that you can live an active, full life without debilitating pain.
• The different types of arthritis, their symptoms and how to alleviate their painful side effects.
• The pros and cons of over-the-counter arthritis medications, plus simple tips that will help you know how to choose the right supplements.
• Free, yet effective ways to get relief from arthritis pain and inflammation, so you don't have to suffer anymore.

the effects arthritis can have significant impact on your physical and mental well-being, but this books shows you how to overcome its painful symptoms and live life relatively pain free.

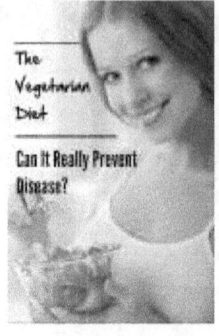

The Vegetarian Diet – Can It Really Prevent Disease?

https://www.createspace.com/5519874

Is a vegetarian diet right for you? Multiple studies have shown over and over that a vegetarian diet goes along way in preventing certain chronic diseases, such as:

• Heart Disease
• Cancer
• Diverticulitis
• Type 2 Diabetes
• Hypertension
• Obesity
• Kidney Failure

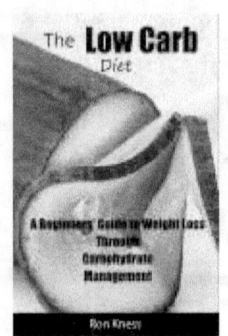

The Low Carb Diet: A Beginner's Guide to Weight Loss Through Carbohydrate Management

https://www.createspace.com/5416348

In my book "The Low-Carb Diet – A Beginners' Guide to Weight Loss Through Carbohydrate Management", I reveal a successful method of losing weight based in part on the amount and type of carbohydrates you consume.

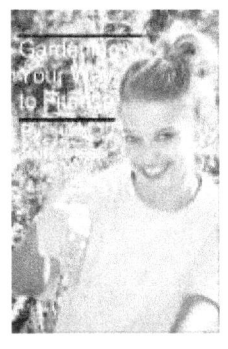

Gardening Your Way to Fitness: The Fun Way to Get Fit and Provide Beauty and Healthful Bounty for Your Family

https://www.createspace.com/5459564

The gym is a great place to stay fit during the colder seasons, but once the temperature turns warmer you want to spend more time outside. Plus, you'll have the benefit of fresh wholesome produce to enjoy by growing vegetables in your backyard garden.

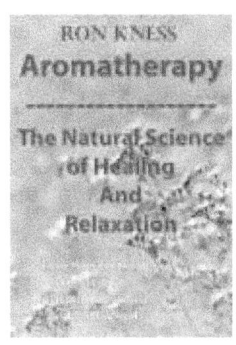

Aromatherapy - The Science of Healing and Relaxation: Learn How Essential Oils Elicit The Relaxation Response And Alter Mood

https://www.createspace.com/5714434

In my book Aromatherapy – The Science of Healing and Relaxation, we reveal the natural holistics methods you can use to heal the body from certain medical issues and to relive stress through relaxation. In particular we talk about:
• Aromatherapy - what it is and how it works
• Essential Oils – how the effects of certain aromas differs from others
• Recipes – how to make your own essential oil combinations

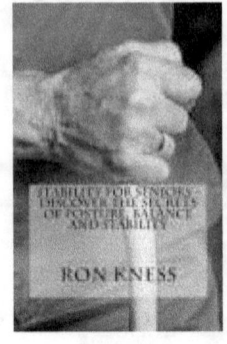

Stability for Seniors: Discover the Secrets of Posture, Balance and Stability

https://www.createspace.com/6096479

Many people sacrifice their health in pursuit of their career. They are so busy making a living that they neglect to make a life. The excuse that they do not have time to exercise is tossed about so frequently that they end up letting their health and fitness slide.

If you are not regularly active, you will have muscular atrophy over time. Your flexibility will decrease. Your core strength will diminish. As time progresses, you will be less limber and more rigid.

This is exactly how people age poorly. It's a process that has snowballed over time.

Only with regular exercise and a healthy diet can you have a body that is fit and has the ability to almost reverse aging.

If you have neglected your health for years and life seems to be a chore now because you can't get around without assistance, do not feel dejected.

You can remedy the situation. You can restore the strength, balance and stamina that you have lost. It is never too late to become what you might have been.

This guide will show you exactly what you need to do to restore your balance, strengthen your core and give you the ability to live life to its fullest. Read how …

About the Author

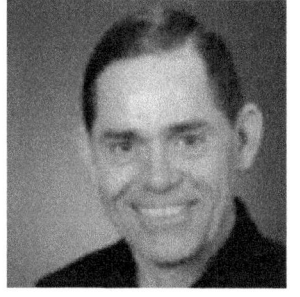

I grew up in Central Minnesota, where my parents own and operated a fishing resort. Once out of high school I tried a couple of semesters of college, only to quit halfway through the Spring term; I decided at that time that college wasn't for me.

Then I decided to follow my father's previous occupation as an auto mechanic. I graduated from a two-year of vocational training course and worked as a mechanic. While in vocational training, I decided to join the National Guard where I eventually ended up working full-time for 32 years.

So how does all of this relate to writing? In one of my leadership schools, the instructor, who was an English teacher at a juvenile detention center, presented writing to me in a whole new way - a way that started to develop my interest in working with words.

Fast forward about 40 years and I now have over 50 books listed on Amazon for Kindle and CreateSpace.